Adrenal Fatigue

Daniel Jackson

Adrenal Fatigue

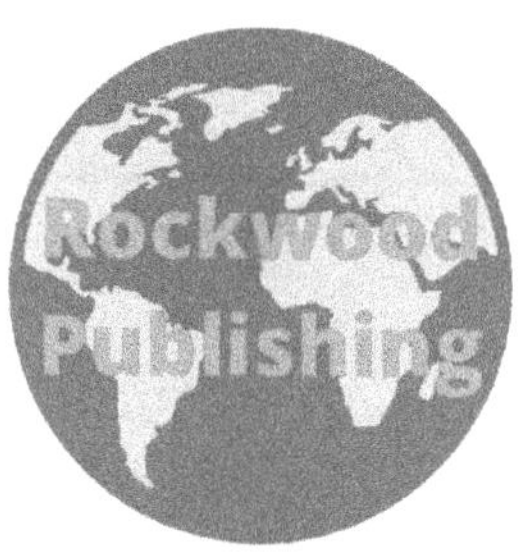

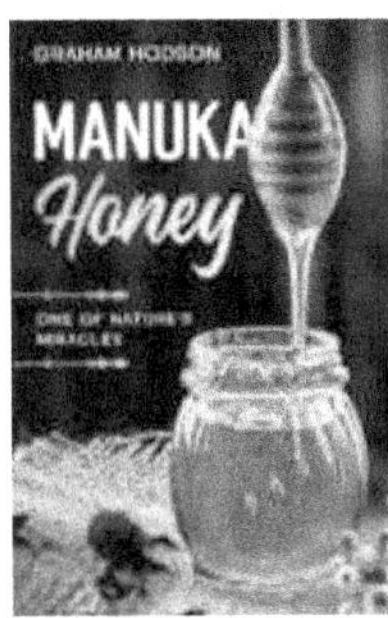
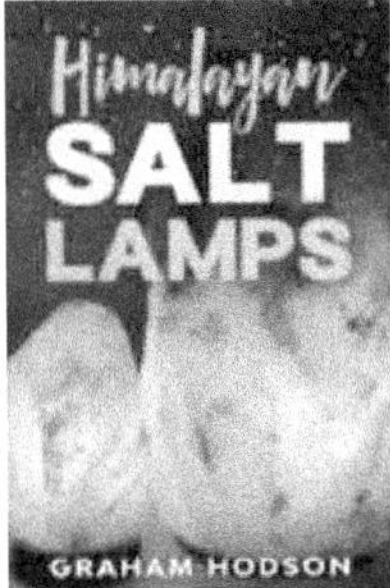
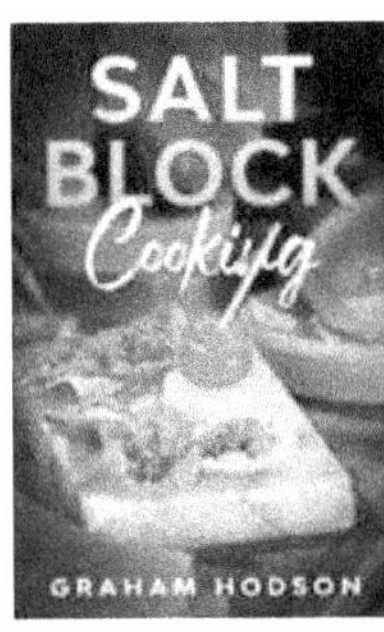
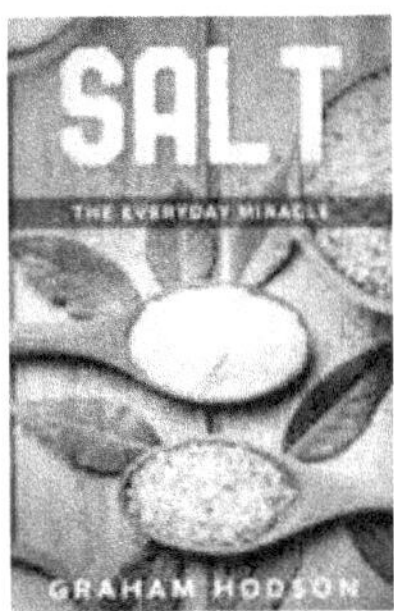
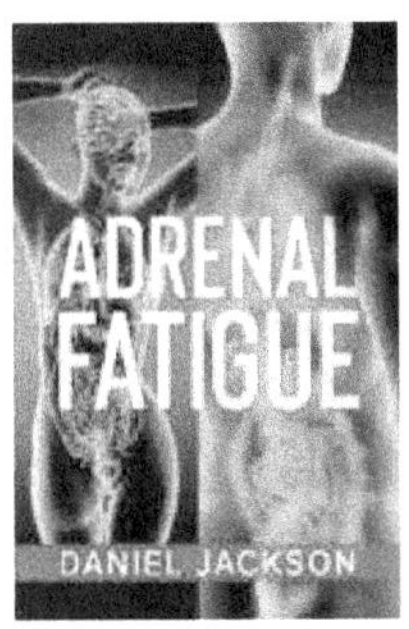
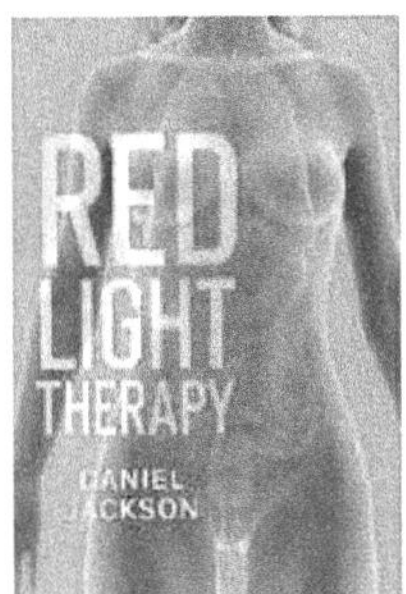
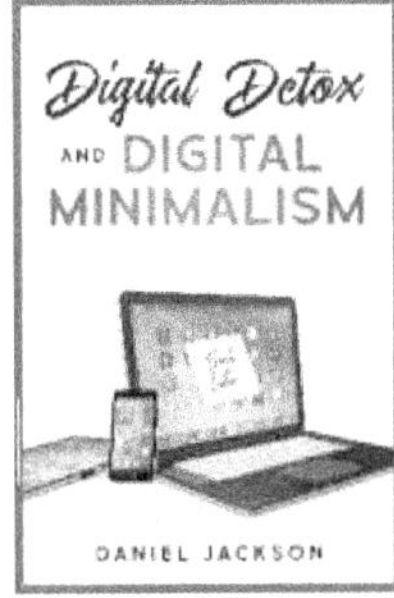
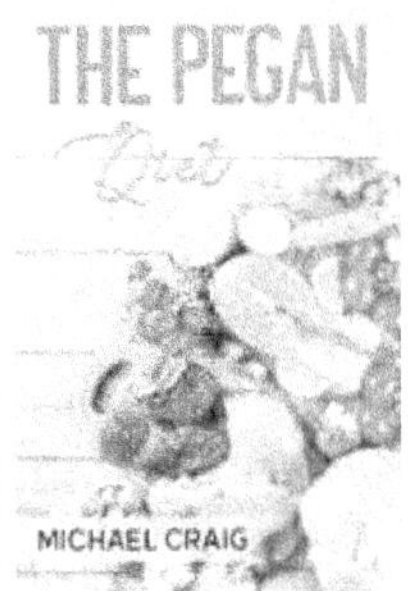

Take a look at more great books available from
Rockwood Publishing

… some for FREE!

Just visit the link below:

rockwoodpublishing.co.uk

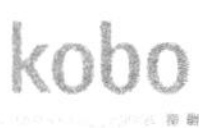
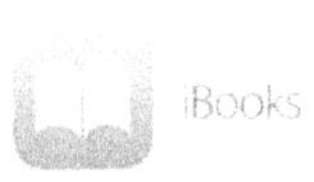
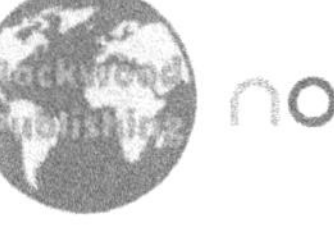
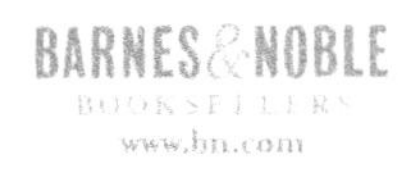

Sometimes the smallest step in the right direction ends up being the biggest step of your life.

Contents

What is adrenal fatigue?

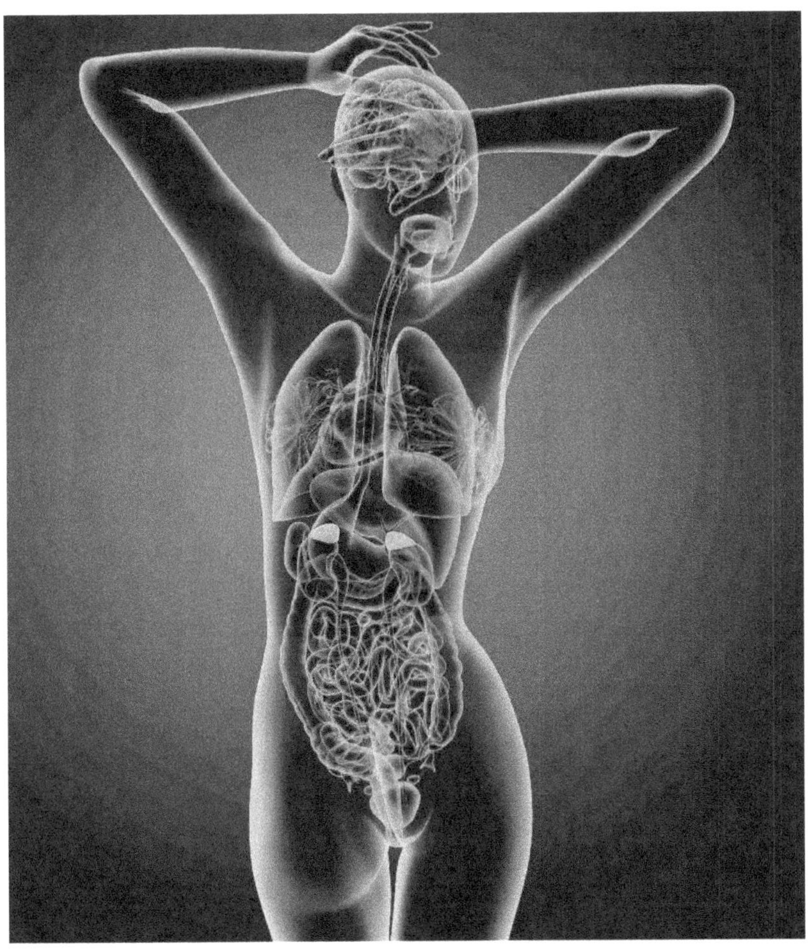

Adrenal fatigue is a generic term that relates to a set of nonspecific symptoms, such as body aches, sleep disturbance, fatigue, nervousness, and certain digestive problems.

The adrenal glands produce many specific hormones that are essential for life.

The medical term "adrenal insufficiency" refers to the inappropriate or inadequate production of one or more of these specific hormones due to an underlying condition or disease.

Adrenal fatigue or Hypothalamic-Pituitary-Adrenal axis (HPA axis) dysfunction is a major underlying cause of many unrelated chronic health problems and is often misdiagnosed.

The symptoms of adrenal fatigue more appropriately refer to the symptoms of the secondary HPA axis, which is your body's collective hormonal response system to chronic stress.

"HPA" refers to three glands that secrete hormones: the hypothalamus and pituitary gland in the brain, and the adrenal glands located above the kidneys.

New, unpredictable, threatening, or uncontrollable situations activate the HPA axis to mobilize the energy necessary to adapt to the demands of the situation.

When your body is repeatedly and continually bombarded by stressful situations and prolonged stress responses, you will eventually pay the price. Your HPA axis may begin to either underreact or overreact to stress, or it may function at inappropriate rates.

This, in turn, is a burden on your body's nervous, hormonal, immune, metabolic, and cardiovascular systems, causing fatigue, insomnia, and a variety of additional physical and psychological symptoms that are generally known as adrenal fatigue symptoms or symptoms of HPA dysfunction.

The Stress Response

When the body receives stimuli of either real or perceived threat, it adapts to these stresses by way of a system called the hypothalamic-pituitary-adrenal axis (HPA axis).

An area of the brain called the hypothalamus responds to possible environmental threats by sending a signal, in the form of chemicals, to the pituitary gland.

The pituitary gland in turn sends its own chemical signals to the adrenal cortex by way of a hormone called adrenocorticotropic hormone (ACTH).

When we are under constant stress, a change in the HPA axis takes place which diminishes the body's ability to adapt to new internal or external stressors.

This leads to adrenal fatigue which can also progress even further to a condition called adrenal exhaustion.

Both conditions however can eventually lead to tissue breakdown, chronic inflammation, and accelerated aging.

The Phases of Adrenal Fatigue

Phase 1 – Alarm Reaction

With adrenal activity, the first stage is called the alarm reaction.

This is where are the system is kicked into action by a stressful situation and reacts by increasing cortisol levels.

This is exactly as it should be. A healthy survival-based response that we all subject our bodies to on a daily basis.

Phase 2 - Resistance

This is referred to as the "resistance stage" and during this phase, the body tries to adapt to chronic, sustained, and prolonged stress.

In order to do so, the body will "steal" pregnenolone from cholesterol so as to make more cortisol, and this action is given the simple and highly appropriate term of, believe it or not, "pregnenolone steal"!

Pregnenolone is central to the formation of sex hormones and when pregnenolone steal occurs, it will lead to the obvious resultant hormone imbalances.

If these imbalances continue over a prolonged period of time it can lead to quite serious hormonal problems such as infertility, PMS, and polycystic ovary syndrome.

Phase 3 - Exhaustion

This final phase of adrenal fatigue is called the "exhaustion phase". This phase is reached when the adrenals have been so stressed and fatigued over time that they are no longer able to adapt to stress.

All the cofactors that are required to make cortisol are used up resulting in a severe drop in cortisol levels, and the pregnenolone steal ceases altogether.

The body has reached the point where it is unable to produce adequate energy.

Fatigue, gut barrier breakdown, blood/brain barrier breakdown, protective skin barrier breakdown, and accelerated aging all occur once you are in this phase.

Conditions related to HPA axis dysfunction

In addition to chronic fatigue syndrome, several other fatigue-related conditions, such as fibromyalgia, post-traumatic stress disorder (PTSD), and depression are associated with stress and a poor HPA axis.

Other conditions related to HPA axis dysfunction and associated with symptoms of adrenal fatigue include:

- Obsessive-compulsive disorder (OCD)
- Panic disorder
- Depression
- Anorexia nervosa
- Chronic and active alcoholism
- Mellitus diabetes
- Central obesity (metabolic syndrome)
- Post-traumatic stress disorder (PTSD)
- Chronic Fatigue Syndrome
- Fibromyalgia
- Premenstrual tension syndrome
- Postpartum period
- Rheumatoid arthritis
- Asthma, eczema (eczema)

Even in people who have no other medical problems, studies have found that if they perceive that they are too stressed, they are much more likely to suffer from increased fatigue, sleep problems, and other symptoms of adrenal fatigue.

For example, studies on work-related stress - caused by overcommitment, lack of social support, high demands, lack of control, and lack of rewards - have been shown to drain energy resources and cause fatigue.

So, it is clear that relentless stress can, and does, have a direct physiological effect on the body. Your HPA axis becomes relatively dysfunctional, and the eventual result is the appearance of symptoms of adrenal fatigue.

General Symptoms of Adrenal Fatigue

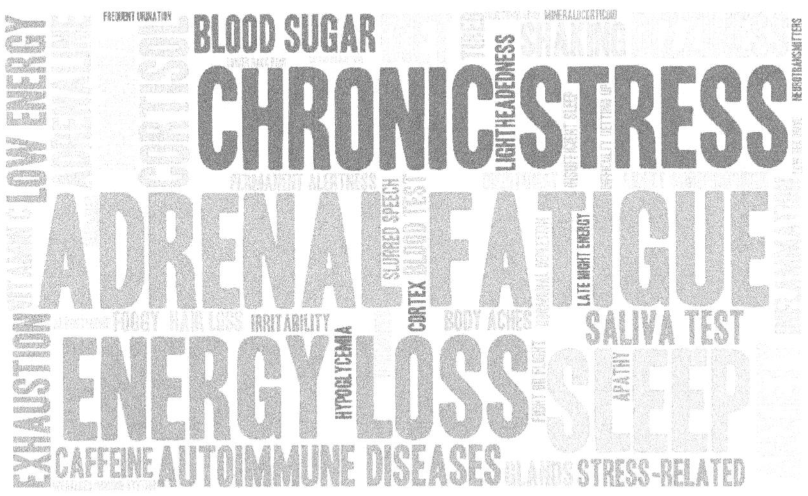

Symptoms of HPA axis dysfunction can include a persistent and excessive feeling of tiredness and a lack of energy that doesn't go away – and this is key - **no matter how much you sleep.**

In addition to the feeling of a general lack of energy, however, adrenal fatigue symptoms can include one or more of the following:

- Weakness
- Muscle pain
- Joint pain

- Throat pain
- Headaches
- Dizziness when standing up
- Increase in cardiac frequency
- Changes in appetite
- Bowel and stool changes
- Abdominal pain
- Depression
- Apathy
- Irritability
- Sleep disorders
- Difficult to focus
- Memory problems
- Confusion
- Anxiety
- Drowsiness

Numerous studies have examined and detailed the relationship between adrenal fatigue, anxiety, stress, HPA axis activity, and fatigue.

People with chronic fatigue syndrome (CFS), for example, very often report significantly higher levels of stress.

In CFS patients, HPA axis dysfunction (characterized by lower-than-normal cortisol secretion) is one of the hallmarks, and studies have shown that the lower the cortisol levels, the more severe the fatigue and other symptoms.

Detailed Symptoms

Sleep and Energy Patterns

a) Power dips in the early afternoon followed by a last-minute energy boost.

b) Usual tiredness at night, but reluctance to lie down. Moreover, later on, feeling wide awake in bed.

c) You feel exhausted in bed, but your head won't stop turning things around and around.

d) Difficulty sleeping. As well as waking up around 2:00 am - 3: 00 am.

e) Severe insomnia

f) Sleeping for long periods (10 hours or more). However, you still have difficulty getting up in the morning.

Sleep and Energy Patterns

a) Anxiety. Often for no apparent reason

b) Panic attacks

c) Depression (mild to severe). If your depression has reached the point where it's having an impact on your life, you should seek professional help immediately

There is so much help and understanding out there these days, and lots of solutions. Nobody has to suffer needlessly anymore.

d) Short-term memory loss and lack of concentration

e) Lack of motivation

f) Pessimism, negative auto-suggestion, or feeling like you cannot trust anyone. It can also present itself as a feeling that nothing is going right or that nothing matters

g) Lack of self-esteem and loss of confidence

h) "Anesthetized" emotions. However, you also find it very easy to cry

i) Slowness and clumsiness of thought

j) Diction difficulties, slurring of words. It may improve after a stimulant like coffee

k) Irritability, anger, tension. In the final stages, it can turn into loud outbursts and arguments at home and/or at work

l) Hypervigilance (very fast reflexes). Getting startled or scared easily

m) Tremors when being in a stressful situation

n) Constant worries

o) Isolation, slight resistance to socializing, avoiding interactions with others

p) Severe lack of patience

q) Tendency to having an addictive nature (smoking, alcohol, online etc.)

r) Nightmares

Digestive and Elimination Symptoms

a) Constipation, usually in the early stages

b) Occasional diarrhoea, especially in the final stages

c) Light beige stools

d) Urinating often, and shortly after drinking

e) Irritable bowel syndrome

f) Bloating, gas, cramps

g) Undigested food

Skin, Hair, Teeth, Bones, Nails, and Muscles

a) Loss of hair on the legs, arms, head, and outer part of the eyebrows

b) The skin looks older than it should for your age

c) You bruise easily

d) Muscle cramps

e) Muscle or lumbar pain

f) Muscle weakness, tired legs when climbing stairs

g) White spots on the nails

h) Bruxism, clenching or grinding your teeth while sleeping

i) Jaw pain

j) Reduction of bone density

k) Neck stiffness

l) Muscle loss

m) Prematurely gray hair

n) Bone-ache

o) Joint pain and stiffness

p) Waking up with numbness in the hands

Dehydration

a) Excessive sweating with little activity

b) Night sweats

c) In general, intolerance to temperatures and low body temperature usually occurs in the final stages

d) Low body temperature

e) Inability to withstand low temperatures. You tend to feel cold even when others don't

f) Cold hands and feet

g) Heat intolerance

Food Sensitivities, Hypoglycaemia, and Cravings

a) Salt craving is experienced at virtually every degree of adrenal fatigue

b) Loss of appetite

c) Exaggerated hunger, hungry even after eating

d) Hypoglycaemia

e) Food sensitivities

f) Craving for chocolate and sweets

Respiratory problems

If you have been in a state of chronic stress for a long time, you'll probably exhibit symptoms of chronic subconscious hyperventilation. These can include:

a) Feeling out of breath

b) Frequent sighs and gasps of air

c) Asthma

Eyes, Ears, Nose, and Throat

a) Sensitivity to light

b) Poor night vision

c) Seeing floating spots in the eyes

d) Blurred vision or trouble focusing

e) Myopia

f) Eye bags

g) Throat pain

h) Tinnitus (ringing in the ears)

Other Symptoms

In addition, you may also experience the following:

a) Lack of libido

b) Dizziness, loss of balance, dizziness when standing up

c) Palpitations, fast heartbeat

d) Dull or sharp pain in the area of the adrenal glands
e) Environmental sensitivities, such as frequent reactions to perfumes, dust, etc.

f) Inflammation

g) Chronic infections

h) Respiratory and skin allergies

i) Fibrocystic mastopathy

Obviously, many of the above symptoms can be, and indeed are, associated with numerous other illnesses, but for that very reason, it's wise to mention the possibility of adrenal fatigue to your healthcare provider and undergo the necessary tests in order to either confirm or eliminate adrenal fatigue as a possible cause for your symptoms.

The three stages of adrenal fatigue

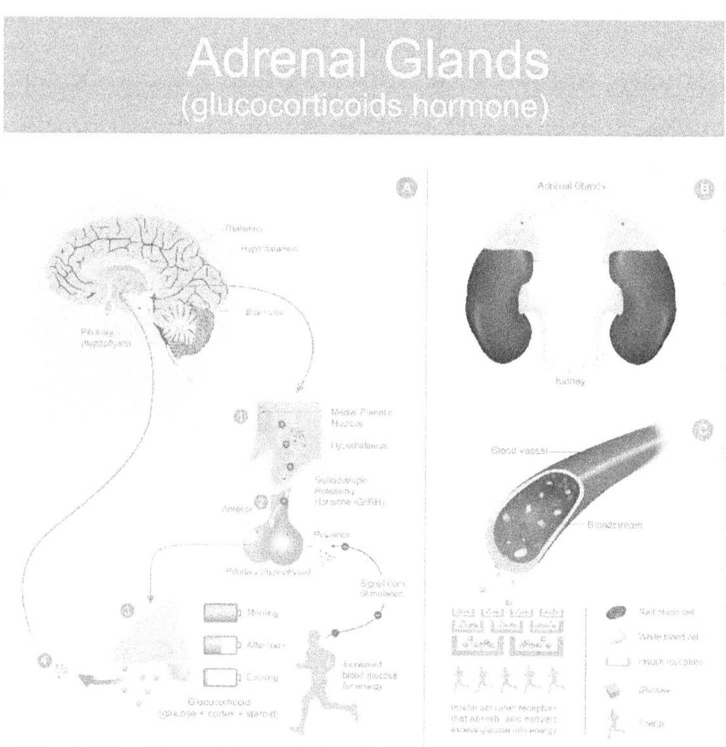

Adrenal fatigue can begin for a variety of reasons, but the basic mechanism behind it still isn't quite fully understood.

Some doctors suggest that it is simply the body's inability to keep up with the production of hormones that are normally manufactured during certain types of stimuli that involve your natural "fight or flight" responses, yet some others believe that it could point to other more serious types of disease.

Recently, studies concerning adrenal fatigue have uncovered contradictory information, making it difficult to pin down the cause exactly, so it's entirely possible that various sets of illnesses and stimuli could trigger events.

Some cases can be caused by something as simple as chronic lack of sleep, or ongoing stress, while other cases may be more difficult to diagnose because the real cause could be stemming from, for example, depression or an autoimmune disease.

As a point of interest, diseases like fibromyalgia are very difficult to detect and are still misunderstood by many health professionals.

While very important pieces of this medical puzzle are still missing, there are quite a few symptoms that most people experience that point to some degree of deficiency of certain essential chemicals in the body.

Blood pressure changes, sudden changes in weight, feeling of restlessness or tiredness, skin discoloration, chronic nervousness, eating or digestion issues, and pain in the extremities or your abdomen are all initial signs that you may have adrenal fatigue.

The three stages of adrenal fatigue are:

1. **High Cortisol Levels** – The usual symptom of this is a feeling of being on edge, while also tired and yet unable to sleep.
   Usually, this causes insomnia, insulin resistance, and weight gain, especially around the middle.

2. **Wrong Cortisol Levels at the Wrong Time** – For example, if you feel constantly stressed and/or tired, or wake up too early in the morning (think 3 to 4 am) and you're unable to go back to sleep.
   People who experience this often have a boost of cortisol just prior to going to bed, resulting in poor quantity _and_ quality of sleep.

3. **No Cortisol Curve** – By this stage, you're completely burnt out. You may even experience

lower hormone levels in other areas as well, such as with thyroid hormones and DHEA.

When you get to this point, you have a much higher chance of developing autoimmune disorders.

Initially, the best way to try and treat any of these issues is with lifestyle changes.

<u>However, don't substitute any of these changes for visits to your doctor in case you have already developed a serious illness.</u>

- **Change Your Diet** – Essentially, you should always aim to eat an inflammatory diet.
  That means that you should rid your diet of gluten, eat clean proteins, and eat lots of vegetables - the more colours the better!

- **Get Sleep** – Train yourself to sleep better.
  Go to bed at the same time every night and get up at the same time every morning.
  Turn off screens a couple of hours before bed and try to sleep at least 7 to 8 hours a night.

Make your bedroom an oasis so that it's calming and easy to sleep in, being sure to keep it cool and as dark as possible.

- **Get Your Vitamins** – A good multi vitamin and multi mineral, Vitamin B complex, D3 and K2, and magnesium.
Some people get benefit from adding vitamin C to their diet too.

- **Improve Inflammation** – Go on an anti-inflammatory diet.
Drink enough water.
Eat plenty of omega-3 fatty acids.
Consider using a curcumin supplement to help further reduce inflammation.

- **Improve Your Nutrition** – When you look at your plate of food, ask yourself whether the items will improve your situation or potentially make it worse.

- **Eat Fermented Food** – Eating foods rich in probiotics can help improve your gut microbiome, which in turn helps your body process nutrients better.

- **Consider a Ketogenic Diet** – For some people, a higher fat diet can improve conditions related to adrenal fatigue while also lessening inflammation. Always seek the advice of a medical professional before embarking on any diet plan.

- **Avoid Caffeine** – While you may be tempted to use caffeine to help with your fatigue, it can be very counterproductive. If you're already addicted, cut down slowly until you fully eliminate it.

- **Avoid Processed Sugar** – White sugar will make your adrenal fatigue worse.

- **Drink Plenty of Water** – The is one of the simplest, yet most effective things you can do. Most people need at least 64 ounces of water per day. If you're exercising or it's hot weather, drink more.

- **Rest Often** – It's best to not overwork yourself if you suffer from adrenal fatigue. Set up your calendar to show everything that needs to be done, for both work and leisure, so that you can plan and pace your days accordingly… and learn to say no!

- **Exercise carefully** – During the first few weeks of treating your condition, as far as exercise is concerned, take it easy. Walk leisurely, gradually working up to 10,000 steps per day. If you can do that without feeling too stretched, you can add other exercises.

- **Learn to Think Differently** – Sometimes it helps if you can change your perception of your situation. Instead of letting it get on top of you, try to turn an initially negative diagnosis into a real positive by making it the catalyst for a better way of life, resulting in you being a healthier person than you were before due to the lifestyle changes you had to make in order to necessitate healing.

Adrenal fatigue may have a lot of non-specific symptoms that could also be related to other illnesses, but they might all be interlinked.

If exposure to stress becomes chronic, the adrenal glands can no longer keep up with the demand, and

DHEA levels begin to decline, signifying adrenal exhaustion.

Also, excess adrenaline secretion can lead you to feel constantly anxious and nervous. Symptoms of insomnia, fatigue, depression, irritability, and digestive difficulties are common.

With adrenaline surges during stress, digestive enzyme secretion is simultaneously lowered, and blood sugar levels rise. As this situation becomes chronic, the combination of high cortisol and prolonged stress adrenaline levels cause, among others:

- A decreased immune function can lead to excessive inflammation and a decreased ability to resist colds and viruses.

- Blood sugar imbalances can lead to a change in appetite, energy, and mental strength

- Increased levels of fat lipids in the blood

- Water retention

- The loss of cellular potassium and, therefore, blood pressure imbalances

- The decrease in insulin sensitivity, with a greater susceptibility to diabetes

- Loss of the ability to make enough DHEA can then lead to changes in the menstrual cycle, sex drive, and fertility

The key to overcoming your adrenal fatigue symptoms lies in breaking the dysfunctional HPA axis cycle, leading the hypothalamus, pituitary gland, and adrenal glands back to balance and to work in harmony again.

This is where natural and holistic approaches shine.

Help maintain your adrenal health with these lifestyle tips

Sleep healthy

It is ideal to be in bed no later than 11 am, even if you feel that during the night is when you are most vital.

Two hours before going to sleep, you should turn off all mobiles, computers, and tablets, as the light they emit (blue light) can block melatonin production, the hormone that regulates the sleep-wake cycle.

In addition, when melatonin is suppressed, cortisol rises, and the natural production of progesterone is interfered with, affecting long-term hormonal balance.

At night, without a doubt, it is better to use dim lighting in the home and full spectrum light bulbs.

Exercise regularly

Like a healthy diet, exercise is vital to our health. It can lower stress hormones such as cortisol, help relax tight muscles, and increase our levels of endorphins - chemicals that give us a sense of well-being.

Walking, swimming, jogging, dancing, or yoga can be excellent types of exercise to relieve stress.

You should avoid demanding exercise if you are going through a very stressful time or suffer from adrenal fatigue since these activities tend to stimulate the adrenal glands even more.

Know the possible causes that generate stress

You should try to identify the main sources of stress in your life. Find what hurts you and eliminate or reduce their occurrence.

Learn to relax

Meditation, deep breathing, yoga, listening to relaxing music, being with "positive" people ... we should look for activities that help us feel more relaxed and/or fulfilled.

Do something that makes you happy

Taking regular time to do something you like and that makes you feel good, or finding a hobby, is essential for psycho-emotional well-being.

Spending time with yourself, without feeling guilty, will do you the world of good. It helps you re-connect with yourself and to "re-charge the batteries".

Laughter, in particular, is a proven reliever of stress, as is surrounding ourselves with the people who make us smile.

Organize your goals and tasks

Good management of your various tasks or projects can lighten your mood and calm your mind.
It is advisable to make separate lists of what you want to do, and what you must do.
Feeling in control and trusting in our potential can reduce stress.

Work and personal life, find balance

Try to avoid thinking about work when you are at home. If we are with the family, take advantage of that wonderful time and definitely don't make them feel "in the way" or that you're, in effect, "absent".

We must value this precious time and separate our work from being with our loved ones or enjoying our hobbies.

Putting yourself first

Before anyone else, there is you.

If we are not well, we can never give the best of ourselves to the rest, and be the best version of ourselves.

Take the time to rediscover your balance and inner peace, feel that you are unique, that you **are** enough, and shine with your light.

Loving and valuing yourself is the first thing you must do.

Don't feel guilty when you "do nothing."

For some of us, this can be a difficult challenge to implement. We live in an age where "doing" is valued more than "being," which can have a detrimental effect on our mental and physical well-being.

Finding time to rest in yourself and just "be" will lead to increased productivity in the long run.

What foods take care of my adrenal glands?

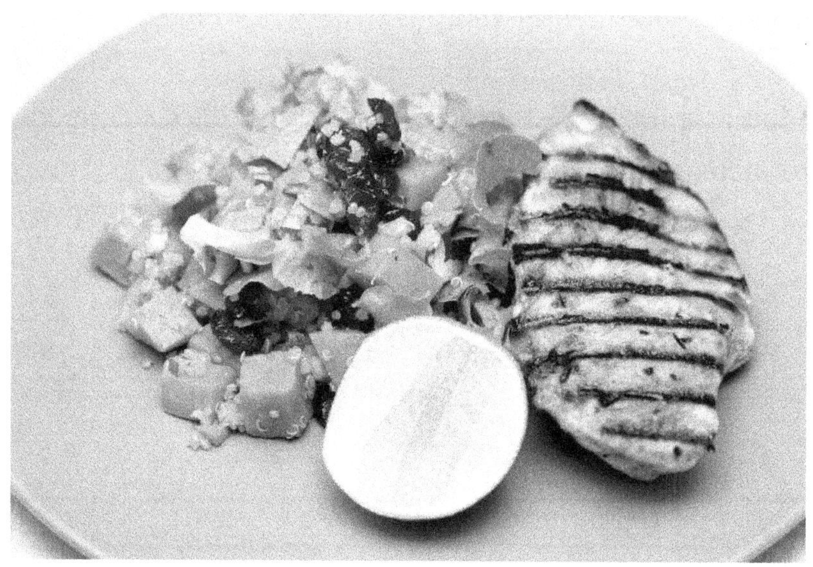

Foods rich in protein

Try to eat protein at every meal. Protein slows down the sudden release of glucose into the bloodstream.

Foods high in protein are eggs (choose organic), meat, fish, legumes (lentils, beans, chickpeas), nuts, seaweed, and seeds.

Dairy products like plain yogurt and cheese are also high in protein, but many people have some degree of intolerance to cow's milk; both intolerances and allergic reactions put more pressure on the adrenal glands.

The best option, depending on the case, is goat dairy products or sheep dairy products.

Alternatively, you can even opt for vegetable kinds of milk and vegetable yogurts.

Foods rich in B vitamins

B vitamins are vital for energy production and the normal functioning of the nervous system. Vitamin B5 is crucial to the production of glucocorticoid hormones (produced in the adrenal glands) such as cortisol.

Some good sources are whole grains, eggs, beans and lentils, a wide range of vegetables, fish, and meats (choose good quality organic meat).

Taking a vitamin B complex supplement can be very helpful.

Foods rich in magnesium

Magnesium is essential for energy production and adrenal hormones manufacture and is quickly depleted when we are stressed.

The best natural sources are nuts and seeds (especially pumpkin seeds and hemp seeds), oatmeal or buckwheat flour (not related to wheat and gluten-free), green vegetables like spinach, crucifers like kale, and fish and shellfish.

Foods rich in vitamin C

Vitamin C is another vital nutrient in the manufacture of adrenal hormones.

Fruits and vegetables are the best sources, but contrary to popular belief, oranges do not have the highest levels; the best sources include bell peppers, kale, broccoli, Brussels sprouts, red cabbage, and watercress.

Vegetables are a better option than fruit since a lot of fruit has high levels of simple sugar, which can lead to sudden rises and falls in blood glucose.

"Relaxing" foods

When we feel nervous, tense, or stressed, we are tempted to turn to "comfort food" which, all too often, has little or no nutritional value.

Well, why not look for healthy foods or drinks that help us feel calm again?

For example, prepare an infusion of rooibos or kukicha tea, together with a handful of nuts such as rich Brazil nuts (high in selenium) or open an avocado and put it on top of a spelt toast with a sprinkling of poppy seeds.

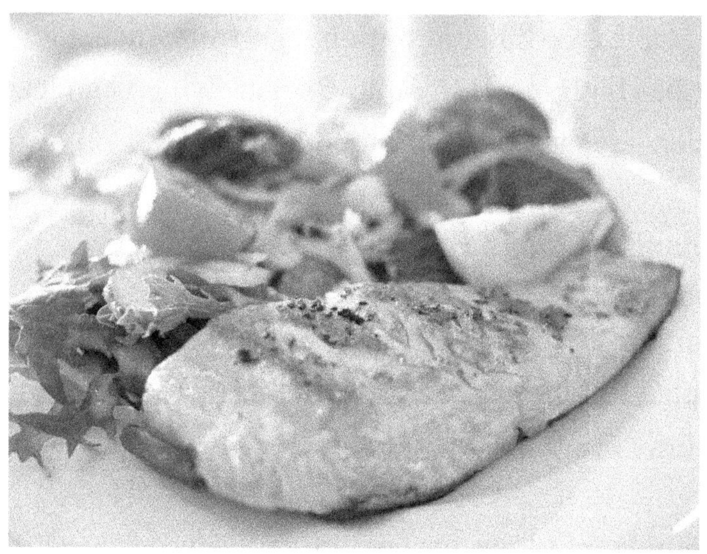

Stress and Illness

In the 1960s, psychiatrists Thomas Holmes and Richard Rahe investigated the impact of different life events.

With the results they obtained, they developed the Holmes and Rahe stress scale.

In it, various events are classified, such as:

- The death of a partner
- Losing your job
- Pregnancy
- Moving home

Each event was assigned a value, with the death of the spouse first, with 100 points. In this way, they discovered that when people reached a certain level of points, they had a high probability of getting sick.

In addition, in their studies, they discovered that stressors are cumulative. Moreover, the greater the exposure to these events, the greater the probability of becoming ill.

So, the takeaway from their studies was that although it obviously isn't possible to go through life without experiencing any stress, it is important to do everything we can to lessen our exposure to stress and, crucially, that we learn how to deal with stressful situations in a way that delivers the best possible outcome with the least possible impact on our body.

A philosophy to which I always try to adhere is simply:

"Act, don't react"

This alone can help with many situations.

How often do we react to something in a split second, only to realise that if we'd merely taken a few moments to actually think about things, we'd have come up with a much better solution for all concerned?

So often when we act on impulse, we end up creating a more stressful situation for ourselves than the stressful event was in the first place!

(Note from the author: don't be harsh with yourself if this doesn't happen every time, because although I always try to "Act, don't react", I have to confess that I sometimes fail. But, hey, we're all only human after all.)

The Renal/Kidney Diet

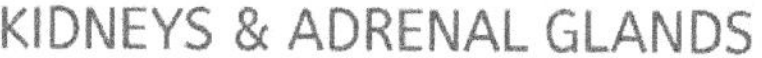

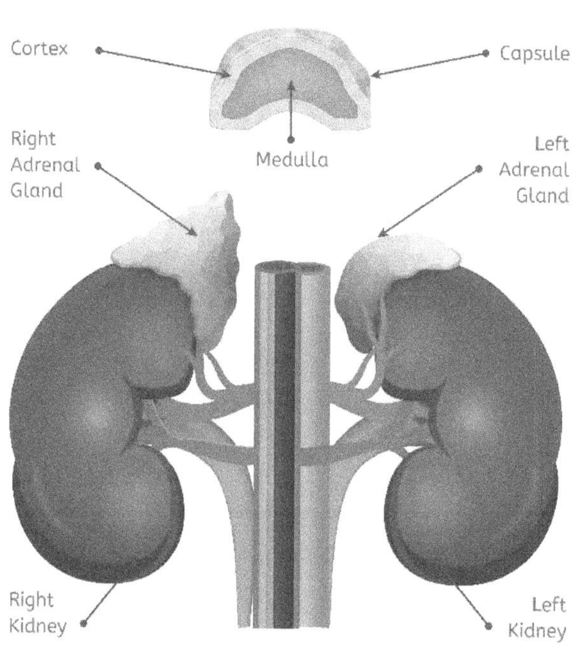

What you eat and drink directly and dramatically affects your health.

For example, staying at a healthy weight and eating a balanced diet with appropriate amounts of salt and good fats can help you control your blood pressure.

Or, if you have diabetes, you can help control your sugar levels by choosing what you eat and drink very carefully.

In the same way, a regime of eating that has become known as the "renal diet" or "kidney diet" can help protect your kidneys from being damaged.
In it, the kidney diet limits certain foods in order to prevent the minerals in those foods from building up in your body.

Kidney diet basics

With all eating plans, including the kidney diet, you need to keep track of the number of certain nutrients you consume, such as:

Calories
Protein
Fats
Carbohydrates

To ensure that you are getting the right amount of these nutrients, you need to eat and drink the right portion sizes.

All the information you need to keep track of your intake is contained in the "nutrition facts" label of the individual products.

The nutrition information will tell you how much protein, carbohydrates, fat, and sodium are in each product and this will help you choose foods rich in the nutrients you need… and low in the nutrients you don't!

Calories

Calories are derived from protein, carbohydrates, and fats in your diet. How many calories you need is determined by your gender, age, body size, and activity level.

You can adjust the number of calories you eat depending on your weight goals.

Some people limit the calories they eat. Others, like high-performance athletes, need to eat more calories.

Your doctor or dietitian can help you figure out how many calories you should be eating each day.

Work with your dietitian to make an eating plan that helps you get the right number of calories, and stay in contact with him/her for support.

Protein

Protein is one of the building blocks of your body.

Your body needs protein to grow, to stay healthy, and to heal when necessary.
Having too little protein can make your skin, hair, and nails weak.
However, having too much protein can also be a problem.

To stay healthy and help you feel better, you may need to adjust the amount of protein you consume.

Some doctors recommend that people with kidney disease limit protein or change their protein source.

This is because a diet that is very high in protein can make the kidneys work harder which could potentially cause damage.

Ask your doctor or dietitian how much protein to eat and the best protein sources for you.

Remember, however, that just because a foodstuff is low in protein does not mean it can be consumed in high amounts.

Carbohydrates

Carbohydrates are the simplest type of energy for your body to use.

A healthy source of carbohydrates includes fruits and vegetables.

Unhealthy carbohydrate sources include sugar, candy, soda, and other sugary drinks.

Some carbohydrates are rich in potassium and phosphorus. We'll discuss this in more detail a little later.

Your dietitian can help you learn more about the carbohydrates in your meal plan and how they can affect your blood sugar.

Fats

You need fat in your eating plan to stay healthy. Fat gives you energy and helps you metabolise certain vitamins in food.

However, too much of certain fats can lead to weight gain and heart disease.

If you feel as though I'm being a little non-committal about dietary fats, you'd be right, as in quite recent times there has been the most breath-taking change of direction from certain sectors of the medical profession concerning fats.

Mainstream doctors are still sticking to the age-old "don't eat saturated fats" narrative, while other sectors have performed a dramatic U-turn which is reminiscent of a 90-mph handbrake turn in the latest Fast and Furious movie!

So, the only thing I can advise here as this book goes to print during a constantly changing and updating stance on fats is for the reader to employ due diligence and thoroughly research the latest guidelines as to the consumption of the different types of fats.

However, you should **always** avoid trans fats found in margarine, fried foods, cakes, and cookies amongst others.

This type of fat makes your "bad" cholesterol (LDL) go up, and your "good" cholesterol (HDL) go down.

When this happens, you may be more prone to heart disease, which is, obviously, serious enough in its own right, but a double whammy in that it can also cause or worsen kidney damage.

Sodium

Sodium is a mineral found in practically all foods. Too much sodium can raise your blood pressure, as can too little potassium.
High blood pressure can damage your kidneys or worsen a pre-existing condition.

It is usually wise to limit and/or monitor your sodium intake.

To limit sodium in your meal plan:

- Do not add salt to your food when you cook or eat. Try cooking with fresh herbs, lemon juice, or unsalted spices.

- Choose fresh (or frozen) vegetables in preference to canned vegetables. If you are using canned vegetables, drain and rinse first in order to remove the salt before cooking or eating.

- Avoid processed meats like ham, bacon, hot dogs or chorizo, and lunch meats.

- Opt for fresh fruits and/or vegetables instead of salt-laden snacks.

- Avoid canned soups and frozen meals that have a high sodium content.

- Avoid pickled foods.

- Limit high-sodium condiments such as soy sauce, ketchup, and barbecue sauce.

Important!
Be wary of salt substitutes and "reduced sodium"
foods as they can be high in potassium.

Although too little potassium can lead to high
blood pressure (because the sodium/potassium
ratio is a crucial and delicate balance), too much
potassium can be dangerous if you have kidney
disease.

Work with your dietitian to find the optimal
balance for sodium and potassium.

Always use a high quality, natural, unrefined salt like
Himalayan salt or Celtic Sea Salt so as to avoid
ingesting talc (found in most commercial table salt)
and plastic particles (found in some sea salts).

For literally _everything_ you need to know about salt, I
strongly recommend you read the book
"Salt – The Everyday Miracle", a real eye-opener of a
book that is available on Amazon.

Portions

Choosing to eat healthy foods is certainly a great start, but remember that eating too much of anything, even healthy foods, can potentially be a problem.

So, an often-overlooked part of a healthy diet is portion control or, put simply, watching just how much you eat.

Check the Nutrition Facts label on all foods as many packages have more than just one serving.

For example, a 20-ounce bottle of soda is two and a half servings.

Fresh foods, such as fruits and vegetables, tend not to come with nutritional information labels, but even they can be consumed in too large a quantity.

Ask your dietitian for a nutrition list of fresh foods and advice on how to measure portions correctly.

Top Tips:

1. Eat slowly and stop eating when you are no longer hungry. It takes about 20 minutes for your stomach to tell your brain that it is already full. If you eat too fast, you may eat more than you need.

2. Avoid eating while doing something else like watching TV or catching up on some work. When you are distracted, you do not realise how much you have eaten.

3. Do not eat directly from the food package. Instead, take out only one portion of food and put the rest away.

Controlling portion sizes is important to any meal plan. It is even more important on a kidney diet because you may need to limit not only what you eat, but also how much you eat.

When your kidneys aren't working as well as they should, waste builds up in your body. After a while, it can cause various health problems.

A kidney diet meal plan can limit the amount of certain minerals you consume. This can prevent waste from building up and causing problems.

How strict you need to be with your plan is dependent on the stage of your kidney disease.

Potassium

Potassium is a mineral that's found in nearly all foods. Your body needs potassium for your muscles to work, but too much potassium can be dangerous.

When your kidneys are not working well, your potassium level can sometimes be either very high or very low which can cause muscle cramps, problems with heart rhythm, and muscle weakness.

If you have kidney disease, then you may need to control just how much potassium you consume. Ask your doctor or dietitian if you should limit your potassium intake.

Your doctor may prescribe a medicine called a potassium binder to help your body get rid of the extra potassium.

Remember, you must always seek the guidance of your professional healthcare provider as far as potassium intake levels are concerned, as although too high an intake can be bad for your kidneys, too low an intake can seriously impact your blood pressure.

Phosphorus

Phosphorus is also a mineral found in almost all foods. It works with calcium and vitamin D to keep your bones healthy.

Healthy kidneys maintain the correct level of phosphorus in your body, but when your kidneys are not working as they should, phosphorus can build up.

Too much phosphorus in your blood can lead to bones breaking easily.

Many people with kidney disease need to limit their phosphorus intake.

It's important to ask your doctor if you need to limit phosphorus.

Depending on your stage of kidney disease, your doctor may also prescribe a medicine called a phosphorus binder.

This can prevent phosphorus from building up in your blood. Although a phosphorus binder can help, you should still watch how much phosphorus you consume in your diet.

Liquids

Our bodies need water to survive, but when you have kidney disease, you may not need it as much. This is because when the kidneys are damaged, they do not remove extra fluids quite as they should.

Too much fluid in your system can be dangerous as this can cause high blood pressure, swelling, and heart failure.
Fluids that build up near your lungs can make it difficult for you to breathe.

Depending on the stage of kidney disease and your specific treatment, your doctor may ask you to limit the amount of fluids you drink.

You may also need to cut out certain foods that have high water content.

Soups, and foods that melt, like ice cream and gelatin, have plenty of water, so you'll need to watch these. Many fruits and vegetables are also high in water content as well.

If you need to limit your fluid intake, drink small amounts and keep track of exactly how much you have been drinking.

Limit the amount of salt you consume so as to avoid thirst.

Special diet concerns

Vitamins

Following an eating plan on a kidney diet can sometimes prevent your body from getting enough of the vitamins and minerals it needs.
To help you achieve the right level of vitamins and minerals, your dietitian may suggest a supplement.

Important! Tell your doctor or dietitian about any vitamins, minerals, supplements, or over-the-counter medications you are taking. Any of these could potentially damage your kidneys or cause other health problems.

Following a kidney diet for diabetes

If you have diabetes, you need to control your blood sugar levels to prevent damage to your kidneys.

Your doctor or dietitian can help you create an eating plan that will help control your blood sugar level while at the same time limiting sodium, phosphorus, and potassium to the appropriate levels.

Effective Ways to Restore Your Energy Levels

Fatigue is without a doubt something that all of us experience from time to time.

It's natural for us to feel fatigued if we engage in something that is physically, mentally, and emotionally stressful.

The body's response to stress is to release hormones that help us deal with stress. These hormones can give us extra speed, strength, and in some cases, make us impervious to pain.

However, if we regularly subject our body to excessive stress, over time our adrenal glands will become affected, leading to an eventual slowdown in the production of hormones.

When this happens, our body is no longer able to deal with stress effectively and efficiently.

With adrenal fatigue, you constantly feel tired and unable to concentrate. Unfortunately, merely sleeping will not get your energy levels back up.

Adrenal fatigue can be caused by various triggers like anaemia, depression, stress, obesity, eating disorders, low blood pressure, and infection.

One way to treat adrenal fatigue and restore your energy levels is by changing your lifestyle, as most people who suffer from adrenal fatigue are people who generally don't get enough sleep, don't exercise, are overly stressed, and/or don't eat the right foods.

NB, It is important to seek medical help if fatigue is sudden or persistent even if you have adequate rest.

Herbs and Supplements to Improve Adrenal Fatigue

The following is a list of nutrients that will help you more effectively adapt to stress resulting in better resistance to developing adrenal fatigue and adrenal exhaustion.

However, it's very important that you don't start taking any supplementation without first consulting your professional health care practitioner.

- Vitamin B5 - Key nutrients for the production of Coenzyme A which is critical for energy metabolism. B5 is used in the production of cortisol and people who have adrenal fatigue further deplete their levels of B5 in order to produce cortisol which can lead to adrenal exhaustion. Also supports mitochondrial activity.

- Vitamin B6 - Vital for the production of serotonin and dopamine which play a central role in sleep and energy levels.

- Vitamin C - Involved in the production and modulation of cortisol and in boosting the immune system

- Magnesium - One of the most important minerals in the body. A deficiency can lead to a lack of production of neurotransmitters and hormones. Up to 78% of the population in industrialized countries are deficient in magnesium. Correct levels can make a massive difference to mood sleep and energy

- Essential minerals - The clue is in the word essential, and these are best derived from wild-caught fish, green leafy vegetables, pink salts, olives, grass-fed meats and butter, fermented food, and vegetable broth.

- Probiotics - There is a strong connection between gut bacterial imbalance and adrenal fatigue.

- Adaptogenic herbs - Called such because they help our body adapt to stress by modulating the body's use of our stress hormones. They include

Siberian ginseng, basil, Rhodiola, ashwagandha, and astragalus among others.

- Amino acids - L-taurine, L-tyrosine, GABA, and L-theanine have all been found to be helpful in the treatment of adrenal fatigue.

Also worthy of note are the following which has been shown to help in the treatment of adrenal fatigue:

- N-acetyl cysteine
- Alpha-lipoic acid
- Antioxidants
- Coenzyme Q10
- Acetyl l-carnitine

4 Types of Adaptogen Herbs for Treatment

When you're facing a potentially frustrating disorder like that of the adrenals, there are a number of helpful natural treatments that you can employ.

One of the most celebrated in the natural medicine world is the use of adaptogen herbs, which are powerful, non-stimulating herbs and plants (with the exception of ginseng, which is mildly stimulating).

If you've been considering adaptogen herbs as a potential treatment for your adrenal fatigue, then you'll be happy to learn about the following four superstars of the herb world.

Ginseng

Ginseng has a small number of stimulants that can help revitalize you. It is known for helping the body to more efficiently metabolize stored energy and helps to improve your endurance.

Ginseng contains a high level of antioxidants and is the perfect agent to help you deal with stress and repair damage done to the body by both hormonal imbalance and free radicals, which are known causes of cancer. It is also an excellent counter to oxidative stress.

Licorice Root

Like many of the herbs on this list, licorice root has the ability to foster a major increase in energy by boosting the immune system, and by protecting organs against damage that can be caused by excessive cortisol.

When cortisol is under control, it is easier to achieve a more balanced emotional state and to improve metabolic functions.

Please remember that while the root has many positive attributes, it should only ever be used under medical supervision because of its ability to cause major changes to your blood pressure.

Reishi Mushroom

There are a few classes of mushrooms that are powerful antioxidants, and reishi mushrooms are pretty much at the top of the list.

These mushrooms boost immune function and have been linked to decreased tumor activity, and many health professionals have begun to seriously research these useful fungi.

Nutritionists have been recommending the addition of certain mushrooms to the diet for many years due to their positive influence on both depression and hormonal imbalances.

Rhodiola

Having been the subject of numerous studies since the 1960s, Rhodiola has been shown to be very useful in the treatment of depression, anxiety, and other issues of emotions.

In one study, it was used to effectively treat stress experienced by pilots and cosmonauts.

Dietary Changes for Managing Adrenal Fatigue

When our body is under stress it puts a strain on our sympathetic nervous system which is the part of our nervous system connected to the "fight, flight, flee, or faint" response. This is completely normal functioning and is a necessary part of life and survival.

However, problems arise when the sympathetic nervous system is called into action too often and for long periods of time as this leads us into a state of what is termed "sympathetic dominance".

When we are exposed to chronic stress, the hypothalamic/pituitary/adrenal (HPA) axis becomes unable to appropriately produce the hormones and we require in order to keep up with demands. Over time, this results in adrenal fatigue and exhaustion.

The flip side of the coin is that when we laugh, relax, enjoy ourselves, engage in deep breathing, show gratitude, and meditate, we stimulate the parasympathetic nervous system.

This is the part of the nervous system that deals with healing and repair processes.

Under normal circumstances, there would be a good balance between the two systems as each one responds appropriately and accordingly to different external stimuli and situations, with the ratio being in favour of parasympathetic dominance so as to enable healing and repairing from life's daily stresses.

However, the reality is that with 21st-century living, we can easily find ourselves under nearly permanent emotional, physical, financial, mental, and chemical stress which all increase activity of the sympathetic nervous system, which, in turn, leads to greater adrenal hormone output.

This will inevitably lead to problems with the adrenals, namely adrenal fatigue and, if the situation isn't remedied, to eventual adrenal exhaustion.

Adrenal fatigue is a difficult and unpredictable disorder that can have you wondering how you're going to feel from one minute to the next.

An important step in dealing with adrenal fatigue is to identify what sorts of behaviors, habits, and foods might be a possible contributing cause to your condition.

Once you have begun to identify some of the major factors, you can begin to make educated adjustments to your lifestyle so as to be proactive in the improvement of your quality of life.

In the following paragraphs, we'll be discussing some basic dietary changes that you can make to help alleviate the symptoms of adrenal fatigue.

Symptoms

Adrenal fatigue can manifest itself in a wide variety of ways.

It can present with vague symptoms like general tiredness, lack of sleep, major weight gain, sudden weight loss, sudden feelings of nervousness or dread, irritability, and many other generic symptoms, both emotional and physical in nature.

These symptoms can be so varied that the only way to know if there is any sort of deficiency is to get a blood test that can reveal whether or not you have lower counts of specific hormones that should be present under normal circumstances.

For such a relatively small structure within the human body, it's incredible the number of functions and processes that the adrenal glands are involved in.

The two main regions of the adrenal glands are the adrenal cortex and the adrenal medulla.
The adrenal cortex is in the outer circumference of the adrenal glands and produces the following three classes of hormones:

1. Mineralocorticoids: in the main, this is aldosterone which maintains correct salt and water ratios

2. Glucocorticoids: predominantly, this is referring to cortisol which is a hormone produced as a result of the stress response and its function is to increase blood sugar and reduce inflammation.

When we are under constant and chronic stress there is a constant high cortisol level which leads to an increase in blood sugar levels and there for weight gain.

The following Is a list of cortisol DHEA functions;

- Inflammation modulation: immune regulations; pro inflammation; and anti-inflammation
- Detoxification capacity: heavy metals; toxins; hormone detox
- Neural tissue health: Memory; learning; sleep and mood
- Metabolism: weight/fat distribution; body composition; protein turnover; mucosal integrity
- Musculoskeletal: bone turnover; muscle integrity; connective tissue
- Carbohydrate metabolism: cell energetics (mitochondria); glucose; homeostasis
- Endocrine function: thyroid; pancreas; insulin; ovarian function

3. Sex hormones: oestrogen, progesterone and testosterone. Also included are the precursor hormones pregnenolone and DHEA.

The adrenal medulla is the inner region of the adrenal glands and produces the fourth class of hormones, namely catecholamines.

Unique within the endocrine system is the fact that the adrenal medulla has Direct communication with the brain. This is so that if the body is under stress, the brain communicates quickly and directly with the adrenal medulla to raise the levels of catecholamines so as to allow the body to react very quickly to the stressful stimulus.

4. Catecholamines: Dopamine, adrenaline, and noradrenaline.

These are all hormones involved in the so-called famous fight or flight response.
(More recently that phrase has been upgraded to being called the "fight, flight, freeze, or faint" response).

These hormones raise blood pressure, heart rate, respiration, and promote heightened awareness as a survival mechanism against danger, be it real or perceived. The problem, however, is that if we are in a constant and chronic state of stress and hyperawareness, then our bodies become worn down and worn out because, from an evolutionary point of view, we were only ever meant to be under stress occasionally and only for very short periods of time.

The world in which we live today tends to put us under constant stress much more than we were designed to withstand and, consequently, many of us are suffering negative health outcomes.

In short, the four classes of hormones produced by the adrenal glands are:

1. Mineralocorticoids: to maintain blood pressure

2. Glucocorticoids: to maintain blood sugar

3. Sex hormones: For growth, repair, and reproduction

4. Catecholamines: to adapt to stress

So, as you can see, they are little guys that pack a big punch and if they aren't operating at the top of their game your health will suffer.

As discussed previously the adrenal glands react to and adapt to stress and also produce hormones necessary for reproduction.

However, reacting to stress always takes precedence over reproduction as surviving in the first place is perceived as a priority. Once our systems are of the opinion that the danger has passed the adrenals then refocus their energy on producing reproductive hormones.

The adrenal glands are meant to deal with stress and indeed they do and can cope very well as long as there's a natural cycle of stress, rest, and adaptation.

However, problems can develop if the rest part of that cycle is out of balance and this happens when the body is under almost constant stress.

This can lead to eventual adrenal fatigue.

The adrenal glands can end up being overstressed by a good number of different lifestyle factors including:

- Blood sugar imbalances
- Nutritional deficiencies
- Gut inflammation
- Food sensitivities
- Autoimmunity
- Infections yeast viral or bacterial)
- Environmental toxins (heavy metals, pollutants, pesticides etc)
- Ongoing emotional and mental stress
- Physical trauma
- Bad posture
- Ligament damage to the spine

How to Do Some Research

Every person is different and as such it's likely that any foods that work for one person might not work for another. This will require you to do your own research at home before, during and after meals.

This means that in the beginning, it's important for you to eat simpler meals with a smaller list of ingredients and different classes of foodstuff.

As you add foods back into your diet, take a note of if and how it affected you.

Once you know exactly which foods caused a negative reaction, be sure to leave them out of your meals and diet in general.

However, sometimes these reactions aren't permanent, because they could be a sign of a different kind of disorder, but always remain patient so that you can deal with your illness effectively.

Supplements That Help with Adrenal Fatigue

If you discover that there *are* certain foods that you feel you should be avoiding in order to gain some relief from the disorder, it does, in turn, raise one very significant and salient question…

"What about the vitamins and minerals that you get from the foods that you will now have to start avoiding?"

This is where you might be wise to venture down the road of supplements.

Supplements

Finding a good, preferably organic, multi vitamin and mineral might be a great way to help keep your nutrition balanced.

Adrenal fatigue is a collection of symptoms that occur when the adrenal glands function below the necessary levels.

Although most commonly associated with intense and/or prolonged periods of stress, it can also arise as a result of respiratory infections such as flu, pneumonia, or bronchitis.

Supplements can be very helpful in reducing adrenal fatigue, particularly products developed with a combination of ingredients to support adrenal function.

a) Ashwagandha may be the most popular herbal supplement for the adrenals. Known as an adaptogen, ashwagandha helps adrenal glands adjust to stress, produce stress hormones when you need them, and stop producing them when you do not.

b) Vitamin C is also essential for adrenal function as it can lower the amount of cortisol, norepine, and epinephrine produced in response to physical stress when taken in adequate amounts.

c) B vitamins have been shown to be useful in the treatment of adrenal fatigue and those who are experiencing symptoms should consult with their healthcare professional about including a

B complex vitamin, with extra B5, in their daily regimen. B vitamins are important for boosting energy levels and can help reduce adrenal fatigue. Vitamins B5 and B12 can help improve adrenal function.

d) Lastly, magnesium is a very important element for optimal adrenal function. Magnesium is essential for many processes in the body, and magnesium deficiency increases anxiety and depression, which can lead to improper adrenal function.

Probiotics

Another supplement you may wish to take along with vitamins and minerals are probiotics which support the growth of important gut bacteria.

You can also get these essential bacteria by way of yogurt, fermented food, and a variety of speciality drinks.

A word of caution

It's important to observe due diligence and exercise caution when taking supplements because the body demands balance in order to heal.

If you take too much of a substance, you could inadvertently throw your body out of balance, which is, obviously, counter to what you are trying to achieve.

Some minerals can even become toxic, so as far as supplements are concerned, be sure to follow the advice of a medical professional as to what and how much you should be taking.

How To Test Your Adrenal Function

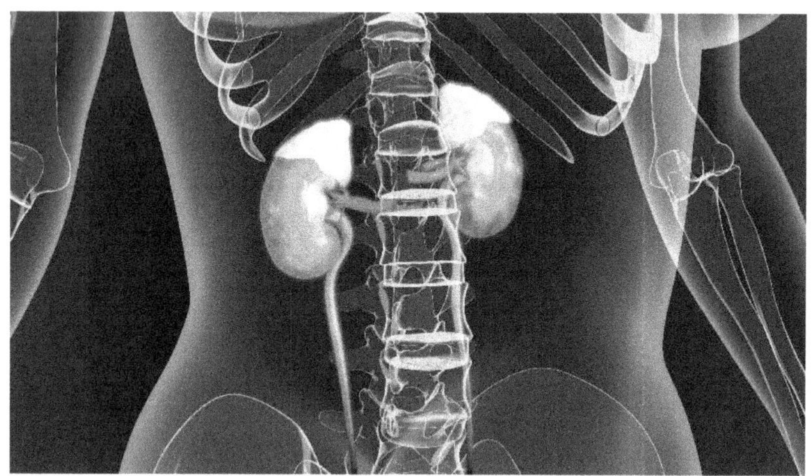

Even though they are each only about the size of a walnut, the adrenal glands produce more than 50 essential hormones, all of which are critical to our health and well-being.

However, when we are overly stressed, the adrenals produce too much of the stress hormones until, ironically, the adrenals *themselves* are fatigued and stressed, leading to an "adrenal crash" or what is known as adrenal fatigue. This is obviously devastating to our body.

There are a variety of symptoms associated with adrenal fatigue, but the most common one is a general lack of energy or inconsistent energy levels.

Adrenal fatigue can be the main cause of certain health conditions; however, it can also be a secondary cause or symptom of another health condition such as upper cervical stress, infections, or blood sugar irregularities.

The actions of the adrenal glands are controlled and coordinated by areas in the brain called the hypothalamus and the pituitary gland.

The connection between these two regions of the brain and the adrenal glands is called the hypothalamic-pituitary-adrenal (HPA) axis.

When the body is placed under constant stress there is a communication breakdown within the HPA axis, sometimes referred to as HPA axis dysfunction, which can result in either adrenal over-activity (adrenal hyperfunction) or indeed under-activity (adrenal hypofunction).

If the individual has an overactive adrenal function, they will produce too much cortisol and will often have increased blood sugar levels which could eventually lead to insulin resistance and diabetes.

Conversely, if they were to have an underactive adrenal function, they will produce too little cortisol resulting in low blood sugar and an increase in inflammation.

The best most accurate way to test your adrenal function is with the previously mentioned DUTCH test, but unfortunately, this can be quite expensive, is really covered on health insurance, and is also a relatively unknown test amongst mainstream doctors as they have rarely ever been trained as to the existence or analysis of this test.

Fortunately, two very simple and inexpensive tests can be performed at home to give an indication as to the possibility of adrenal fatigue.

1.   Blood Pressure

The first is a simple blood pressure test because the adrenal glands play a major role in maintaining normal blood pressure.

People with adrenal hyperfunction (overactive adrenals) will produce high levels of stress hormones and have higher blood pressure, while those with adrenal hypofunction (underactive adrenals) will produce too few stress hormones resulting in low blood pressure.

So, if during your next routine medical examination, you exhibit signs of high blood pressure, it might be worth asking your health professional about the possibility of these higher readings being caused by adrenal dysfunction.

This could potentially avoid being put on blood pressure medication for what could be the rest of your life if you are able to normalise your blood pressure by sorting out your adrenal functions.

It's certainly at least worth asking your doctor and raising this possibility.

2. **Pupillary Constriction Test**

The second simple at-home test for adrenal function is the pupillary constriction test whereby the iris in the eye is tested as to its response to light exposure.

This test works on the premise that individuals suffering from adrenal fatigue are very often unable to maintain the level of contraction of the pupil for a specific length of time.

The test is performed in the following manner:

A. Sit in front of a mirror in a dimly lit room
B. Shine a (not too bright) torch at a 45-degree angle into your eye (i.e., from the side of your face)

And that's it, but as you'd expect, it's what happens when you perform this test that is of relevance.

The pupils of your eyes will naturally constrict when light is shone into them, meaning that their diameter will reduce in size due to the activity of the muscles in the iris (which is the coloured part of the eye).

These are the results to look for:

i) Normal adrenal function (healthy HPA axis) - Pupil remains constricted (smaller) for 20 seconds or more

ii) Mild adrenal fatigue (mild HPA axis dysfunction) - Pupil remains constricted for only 10-20 seconds

iii) Adrenal fatigue (HPA axis fatigue) - Pupil remains constricted for only 5-10 seconds

iv) Adrenal Exhaustion (HPA axis failure/exhaustion) - Pupil will constrict then immediately dilate (go larger) again

Blood analysis

In addition to the above two "at home" tests, a simple but comprehensive blood test via your health provider can reveal a lot about the functioning of your adrenal glands.

Adrenal overactivity (hyperfunction) markers in the blood can include:

- Sodium - high normal or high
- Potassium - low
- Chloride - high
- Blood glucose - high
- Cholesterol - high

Adrenal under-activity (hypofunction) markers in the blood can include:

- Sodium - low
- Potassium - high normal or high
- Chloride - low
- Blood glucose - low
- Cholesterol - low (but possibly with high HDL)

As stated above, people with adrenal dysfunction may exhibit issues with the ratio of sodium to potassium, one of many potential electrolyte imbalances.

To help remedy this, it's important that they adopt a diet that is rich in minerals, and eat foods such as:

- Nuts
- Seeds
- Mushrooms
- Shellfish
- Dark chocolate/cocoa powder
- Whole grains
- Cruciferous vegetables
- Organ meats (organic)
- Beef
- Lamb
- Eggs
- Beans
- Lentils
- Tofu
- Cocoa
- Avocados
- Salmon (wild-caught, NOT farmed)
- Berries
- Yoghurt
- Cheese
- Sardines
- Spirulina

- Vegetable
- Fruit
- Leafy greens

So, in conclusion, in order to test for adrenal function and adrenal fatigue you can:

1. Perform an at-home blood pressure check
2. Perform an at-home pupillary constriction test
3. Have a comprehensive blood test done to check for all markers, levels, and indicators
OR
4. Have a DUTCH test (explained below)

The DUTCH Complete Hormone Panel

The DUTCH (acronym for Dutch Urine Test for Complete Hormones) test gauges adrenal health by measuring DHEA and cortisol levels throughout the course of a day to give an idea as to how well or not your adrenal glands are functioning and responding in an appropriate manner.

In a healthy individual, they would have elevated cortisol levels in the morning and low cortisol levels at night. people with insomnia very often demonstrates this the other way around with high cortisol levels at night resulting in their insomnia but low cortisol levels in the morning leaving the subject feeling very lethargic.

Other people may exhibit cortisol dysregulation whereby there are real ups and downs in cortisol levels throughout the day, rather than the desired steady decline in levels from morning to evening.

Using the above DUTCH system of measuring levels of cortisol and DHEA (amongst other markers), a detailed method of understanding and evaluating the level of adrenal fatigue has been created using a seven-phase model (Phase 1; 2; 3A; 3B; 3C; 3D; 4) which is a much more in-depth assessment than the three-phase system as previously mentioned.

This seven-phase assessment model is explained in detail in the next section.

The 7-phase assessment system

Phase 1: Initial alarm reaction

Minimal fatigue
High cortisol
High DHEA

Normal response to stress often noticed in healthy people who work hard and athletes in training.

Phase 2: Deep alarm reaction

Mild fatigue.
High cortisol
Normal DHEA

At this point, we begin to notice symptoms.

Phase 3A: Resistance stage

Moderate fatigue.
High cortisol
Low DHEA

This is where pregnenolone steal takes place leading to major hormonal imbalances typically marked by insulin resistance.

Phase 3B: Deep resistance stage

Moderate + fatigue.
Low cortisol
Low DHEA

At this stage, the adrenals are so overwhelmed and exhausted that they are beginning to lose the ability to have control over stress.

Phase 3C: Non-adaptive adrenal exhaustion

Severe fatigue.
Low cortisol
Normal DHEA

The pregnenolone steal is now failing to produce enough cortisol.

Phase 3D: Inappropriate DHEA

Extreme fatigue.
Low cortisol
High DHEA

Cortisol levels are very low and the subject may be exhibiting major hormone imbalances and insulin resistance.

Phase 4: Full exhaustion

Bedridden.
Very low cortisol
Very low DHEA

At this stage, both cortisol and DHEA levels are very low and the adrenal glands have completely lost the ability to adapt and react to stress. The subject will more than likely experience blood sugar imbalances at this stage.

Nutrition and Adrenal Fatigue

Nutrition plays a major role in both the development of and healing of adrenal fatigue. As societies, most in developed countries consume far too many carbohydrates, mainly from refined bread, pasta, and rice, and the long list of over-processed junk food.

This leads to blood sugar imbalances and the adrenals have to work extremely hard to try and maintain the stability of blood sugar levels which, understandably, pushes the adrenal glands to the limits... and beyond.

The best way to start rectifying adrenal fatigue is by stabilizing your blood sugar levels.

You can go a long way towards achieving this by using what is termed "good fats" which include organic coconut oil, avocados, and olive oil, grass-fed butter, organic animal products, ghee, and organic coconut milk.

In addition, you'll need trace minerals and phytonutrients from non-starchy vegetables such as celery, cucumber, kale, spinach, radishes, broccoli, and cauliflower.

Also, try to get as many herbs into your diet as possible which should include rosemary, thyme, turmeric, ginger, oregano, and basil.

Antioxidants, which also reduce stress on the body and, therefore, on the adrenals, should be obtained by consuming low glycaemic fruits such as lemons, limes, berries, and apples.

An extremely important component of the diet is what is termed "clean protein" which should be consumed in the form of organic (this is vital) beef, chicken, turkey, wild-caught fish (NOT farmed fish) and if desired, wild game.

In addition to the above, I recommend consuming green tea, fermented vegetables, apple cider vinegar, and, my personal favorites, garlic and onions.

These are all anti-inflammatory foods, and seeing that inflammation causes a great deal of stress on the body, it makes perfect sense that by reducing inflammation you will, in turn, ease the workload of the adrenals.

On the other hand, all pro-inflammatory foods will increase the workload on the adrenals.

These include all products from refined grains such as white bread; factory reared grain-fed meats and eggs; junk food; sugary, carbonated sodas; all deep-fried food and most packaged foods; margarine (which contains trans fats); and processed vegetable oils such as corn oil, safflower oil, and sunflower oil.

18 ways to help recover from adrenal fatigue

1. Keep your magnesium, B vitamins, and zinc levels all within an optimal range.

This can be achieved by eating organic meat products, green leafy vegetables, and pumpkin seeds.

2. Sleep

Oh, my goodness, is there anything that isn't impacted by the quantity and quality of your sleep? This subject could be a book in its own right, but the bullet points are:

i) Get to bed between 10:00 pm and 11:00 pm - this has been discovered to be what's called the "Goldilocks hour" for sleep. Going to bed either before or after this is not good for your body systems.

ii) Sleep for between 7.5 and 8.5 hours per night

iii) Keep your room cool

iv) Have your room as dark as possible - this is good for your circadian rhythm and the depth and quality of sleep.

v) Don't <u>ever</u> have your mobile/cell phone near your head - EMFs stimulate brain activity

vi) Don't have any tech devices in your room

vii) Turn off the Wi-Fi before going to bed

viii) Don't look at any tech screens for at least 1.5 hours before going to sleep - the blue light emitted by device screens suppresses the production of melatonin, a hormone vital for sleep.

ix) Avoid caffeine within 7 hours of sleep

x) Exercise - but only during the day, not at night before bed… and DON'T overdo it as that puts even more stress and strain on the adrenals.

xi) Don't eat within 3 hours of going to bed

In addition to the above, you may also wish to try meditation, gratitude, or mindfulness before bed.

A lot of people enjoy reading before going to sleep, but be sure that it doesn't stimulate your brain as that would be counter-productive.

3.   Anti-inflammatory diet

As discussed above

4.   Deep breathing

The average person takes between 12 and 18 breaths per minute, quite often breathing through their mouth and using only the upper part of their chest. It has been shown in countless studies that shallow breathing like this stimulates the sympathetic nervous system which is responsible for the stress response, putting a heavy load on the adrenals.

To counter this, take time each day to breathe deeply in through your nose for a count of 4, being sure to breathe into your belly (you should be able to see your stomach push outwards) and then slowly out through your mouth for a count of 8 as your stomach slowly goes back in again.

Nasal breathing produces greater amounts of nitric oxide, and belly breathing stimulates receptors located in the lower lobes of the lungs that are linked to the parasympathetic (relax and repair) nervous system.

It has been shown that exhaling for longer than inhaling also stimulates the parasympathetic nervous system.

Aim for between 5 and 6 breaths per minute when doing this simple mindful breathing technique.

5.   Keep moving

Don't sit for too long at a time as this has been proven to put a strain on your body, increasing the inflammatory response and so putting more strain on the adrenals.

6.   Keep your body well hydrated.

It's a little-known fact that when you are dehydrated you stimulate stress hormone production. Drink filtered water if at all possible.

7.   Engage in Grounding or Earthing

These days, due to mobile phones, Wi-Fi, and smart devices, we live in a smog or soup of electromagnetic frequencies (EMFs).

They have been shown to increase inflammation levels and, indeed, to interfere with neurotransmitter functioning.

To counter this, we should engage in walking barefoot on grass, soil, or sand on a daily basis as it has been proved that doing so reduces inflammation, fatigue, and pain, thus reducing strain on the adrenals.

8.   Avoid sugar as much as possible and reduce your caffeine intake to a minimum.

This is fairly straightforward logical. We have already discussed the effects of sugar on the adrenals and it's a well-known fact that caffeine is a stimulant, kicking the adrenal glands into action once again.

9. Listen to gentle classical or meditative music

This stimulates the production of endorphins and serotonin.

10. Visualisation

Use positive visualisation of yourself being calm and well

11. Chiropractor treatment

Vertebrae that are out of alignment can press on nerves that in turn overstimulate the sympathetic nervous system which causes an increase in stress hormone production.

12. Gut Health

A major cause of adrenal fatigue is problems associated with the gut. If you have a healthy gut due to a healthy gut microbiome, you'll put less strain on your adrenals.

13. Make time to relax and play

Self-explanatory

14. Engage in digital minimalism and a digital detox

I have written a book on this subject ("Digital Detox and Digital Minimalism" available on Amazon) that includes many tips on how to lessen your dependency on tech and so reduce your exposure to harmful EMFs

15. Meditate and/or pray and/or be grateful

All the above activities have a hugely calming effect and reduce the production of stress hormones, stimulate the release of endorphins, and engage the parasympathetic nervous system

16. Laugh

It's been scientifically proved time and time again that laughter reduces stress hormones and increases the "happy" endorphins which will, in turn, reduce the load on the adrenal glands. So, the old saying has been right all along - laughter really is the best medicine!

17. Stretch

Tai Chi, yoga, and qigong all help to calm the mind and the adrenals, particularly when coupled with correct breathing techniques, due to the release of endorphins and activation of the parasympathetic nervous system.

18. Sun exposure/Vitamin D supplements

The sun stimulates the production of Vitamin D in the skin and increases the ability of our mitochondria to produce energy (by way of the absorbed biophotons) thus reducing overall stress on the body systems in general.

If you live in a cold climate, take a good quality VitaminD3 and K2 supplement. Take with a source of fats as D3 is a fat-soluble vitamin.

Massage and chiropractic therapy

A seldom considered or often underestimated therapy in the treatment of adrenal fatigue is the use of massage and chiropractic therapy.

Prolonged stress on the body can lead to subluxation, which is the physical compression and eventual irritation of any number of spinal joints and nerves.

This in turn leads to an imbalance between the sympathetic and parasympathetic nervous systems, whereby the former is activated in dominance to the latter.

The sympathetic nervous system is responsible for activating the adrenal glands, so it's easy to see how muscle tightness can adversely affect the adrenals.

In addition, the heavy use of laptops and cell phones/mobiles very often leads to poor posture and all the considerable spinal and neck problems associated with them, particularly what has become known as "tech neck", in which the vertebrae in the neck become, over time, compressed or out of alignment which puts even more strain on the body.

A good chiropractor will restore the correct structure and alignment of the vertebrae which will take pressure off the nerves of the neck and/or spine.

A massage reduces bodily stress in general which increases parasympathetic tone thus taking pressure off the adrenals.

Both chiropractic and massage interventions can be of great benefit for those dealing with adrenal fatigue.

Adrenal Fatigue and COVID-19

From very early on in the COVID pandemic, it was apparent that the disease had multi-organ and multi-system involvement, and can certainly easily knock out the host's stress response, and patients with COVID-19 can undergo structural adrenal gland changes during the course of the illness.

It's also possible that undiagnosed primary and secondary adrenal insufficiency could be a contributory factor in the severity of illness associated with COVID-19 in some patients.

Therefore, it is vital that if you are already suffering from adrenal fatigue or adrenal insufficiency that you inform the physician treating you for COVID-19 as to your pre-existing condition as it could greatly affect your treatment and, therefore, subsequent outcome.

Studies on the SARS-CoV-2 virus outbreak of 2003 (SARS = Severe Acute Respiratory Syndrome), which is the virus that causes COVID-19, revealed that 40% of patients were diagnosed with hypocortisolism more than three months after recovery, and a significant number of that group (approx. 25%) continued to experience adrenal insufficiency for over twelve months, necessitating the administration of hydrocortisone.

The COVID-19 virus uses what's called a "spike protein" on its surface as a means to bind to a type of receptor called an ACE2 receptor. ACE2 receptors are present on many different tissues including those of the heart, lungs, liver, blood vessels, gastrointestinal tract, and in relation to this book, the kidneys. They are also present in the linings of arterial blood vessels (carrying oxygen-rich blood) and venous blood vessels (carrying oxygen-diminished blood), such as those found in the adrenal glands.

One of the theories behind why COVID-19 affects the adrenals is that the cytokine storm caused by this coronavirus results in negative feedback toward the previously discussed hypothalamic-pituitary-adrenal axis which, in turn, can lead to primary or secondary adrenal fatigue or adrenal insufficiency.

So, once again, be sure to discuss the possibility of adrenal insufficiency and its subsequent treatment with your health care provider if you've ever been diagnosed with COVID-19.

Although the lungs are undoubtedly the primary site of injury from COVID-19 which increases the risk of acute respiratory distress, its full range of potential to infect and affect other organs is still unclear, but, nonetheless, evidence is mounting that there is a clear link between COVID-19 infection and it's potential to affect the adrenals, leading to adrenal insufficiency both as a presenting symptom and as a possible symptom of what is termed "long covid".

The adrenal glands themselves can be infected by many different pathogens including bacteria, fungi, parasites, and, relative to this discussion, viruses which can all cause actual structural damage.

In the case of viruses such as COVID-19, disruption to the adrenals can come via an indirect route in so much as antibodies produced by the host against the virus also, rather unhelpfully, attach to the hosts own ACTH (Adrenocorticotropic hormone) which is a hormone produced in the pituitary gland, thus affecting the aforementioned HPA-axis which is vital to proper adrenal function. ACTH controls the production of cortisol, so low ACTH means lower than optimal cortisol levels.

As an unpleasant irony, one of the symptoms of low cortisol is a reduction of the ability to fight infection, the very thing you need to be working at its best when trying to battle COVID.

It has been found that treatment with corticosteroids can help patients with adrenocortical insufficiency by regressing this imbalance and providing the corticosteroid levels necessary to fight infection.

As far as long covid is concerned, a study took place looking at patients who had recovered from COVID-19 and found that three months after recovery almost half of the patients had what is known as "hypocortisolism", that is, low levels of cortisol and the majority of those also had low ACTH levels.

They did find that these low levels of serum cortisol were only temporary, and resolved themselves in two-thirds of the patients within 12 months.

There have been a few cases reported whereby COVID-19 has caused adrenal haemorrhage, due to the vascular structure of the adrenals, as well as endothelial damage and vascular thrombosis, so much so that informed physicians should be on the lookout for, and suspicious of, adrenal insufficiency in patients presenting with COVID-19 along with hyponatremia (abnormally low levels of sodium in the blood) and hypotension (abnormally low blood pressure).

Also, under autopsy, COVID-19 has been found in the adrenal glands and pituitary glands of patients who have, sadly, died from the virus, further suggesting that those organs are "targets" for the disease and, as such, should be high on the index of investigation of any physician treating COVID patients.

A study of 85 peer-reviewed papers looking specifically at the connection between the adrenal glands and COVID-19 has taken place focusing on three distinct phases of covid infection, that is:

1. Active infection phase
2. Post-infection phase
3. Long-term recovery phase

Active Infection Phase

The study concluded that during the active infection phase, the adrenal glands are actually one of the most heavily affected systems in the body in those patients who had Covid-19 infection severe enough to require hospitalization.

It was found that supplementation with the steroid "dexamethasone" served as one of the best and most powerful lifesaving treatments.

Post Infection Phase

The study also found that physicians should be aware of closely monitoring the potential development of adrenal insufficiency following all cases of COVID-19 hospitalisation.

Happily, cases of mild to moderate COVID-19 infection appear in general to have little, if any, effect on adrenaline related hormone production.

However, it is always worth keeping the idea of potential adrenal insufficiency in the back of your mind just in case you feel that you aren't getting better post-COVID infection either quickly enough or to the proper degree and to discuss such a possibility with your health care professional.

Long-term Recovery Phase

Some people who've recovered from COVID-19 experience prolonged symptoms, which has been tagged as "Long Covid".

A few studies have directly addressed the possibility of adrenal dysfunction and adrenal insufficiency as a concern in the long-term recovery from COVID-19, and studies that include adrenal function screening as part of the monitoring of COVID survivors post-infection have shown a large percentage of patients with less than optimal cortisol secretion when undergoing a test called the "ACTH stimulation test", further indicating the need to keep a close eye on adrenal fatigue and adrenal insufficiency in the weeks and months following infection.

In short, the study concluded that adrenal insufficiency might well be a long-term consequence of COVID-19 infection. This could well be secondary to pituitary gland inflammation (hypophysitis) or as a direct result of hypothalamic damage.

It is also recommended that all COVID-19 survivors undergo long-term follow-up so as to exclude any possibility of gradual and/or late-onset adrenal insufficiency.

A significant number of patients who go on to recover from COVID-19 experience the prolonged effects of Long-Covid.

The main symptoms are: fatigue, brain fog, muscular pain, dizziness, joint pain, and cognitive dysfunction that persist three months or more after recovery from the initial symptoms of COVID, shown by consecutive negative COVID tests.

All routine lab panels for inflammation, anemia, thyroid function, liver function, and salivary cortisol can be conducted.

All tests can be negative, *except* the salivary cortisol test which could show very low levels of free cortisol.

This means that Long Covid symptoms could be explained by the involvement of the adrenal glands and possible adrenal fatigue and insufficiency.
Also, it means that measuring the levels of salivary cortisol is an effective method for establishing the correct recovery plan.

In other words, if you've had COVID, keep an eye on your adrenals!

In A Nutshell

The takeaway from this is that, from the point of view of your adrenals, COVID-19 needs careful consideration from two distinct points of view:

1. If you already have adrenal fatigue ***prior*** to infection with COVID, let the physician who's treating you for COVID know about your adrenal condition, as it could

2. be classed as a comorbidity, and will certainly affect what treatment/medication you receive.

3. If your adrenals are in good order, but *then* you get COVID-19, keep a very close eye on your adrenal function both during and, in particular, after you recover from COVID, as there is documented evidence that the adrenals take a real hammering from the virus, either directly or indirectly, and you could end up suffering unnecessarily from Long Covid due to the resulting malfunctioning and inappropriate response of the adrenal glands.

Please don't assume that your COVID physician will automatically check and keep an eye on your adrenals, because they more than likely won't.

It's not that they're being lazy or incompetent, they're not in any way, it's simply that the vast majority of doctors haven't been told about the connection between COVID-19 and the adrenals and adrenal insufficiency.

Don't let yourself fall victim to this either during treatment or afterwards, and do take responsibility for your own health and well-being by asking questions and making sure that you receive full, correct, and appropriate treatment protocols.

You deserve only the very best, so don't make the mistake of leaving it to chance.

In Conclusion

I sincerely hope that you've enjoyed reading this book and that you gained valuable information in connection with the adrenal glands and their dynamic effect on your overall health and wellbeing.

As you've read, they are central to your quality of life and when they are malfunctioning or, to be more precise, under-functioning then, boy, do we know it!

The human body is very often thought about as bone, muscle, blood, skin, and organs etc., but a sometimes-overlooked aspect are the roles of electrical impulses and chemicals, mainly in the form of hormones.

When our hormone levels are in balance, it goes a long way towards good physical health and quality of life.

However, when they're off-kilter, we pay a big price.

It's not only hormones associated with the adrenals that, when out of balance, can greatly diminish our levels of health.

For example, a little-known aspect of child-birth is that for an alarmingly high number of women, their hormone levels never return to normal after giving birth.

They can experience post-natal physical and emotional problems of varying degrees, from very mild to extremely debilitating, and for different lengths of time, from a few weeks to decades, and even for the rest of their lives.

The body has to make changes to certain hormone levels during pregnancy, and in the ideal world, those hormones return to their pre-pregnancy levels after childbirth, but for all too many women, that just doesn't happen.

And yet a simple hormone screening test after a period of time will tell you and your doctor exactly which hormones are at the correct levels and which, if any, haven't returned to normal. Corrective measures can then be taken and potentially years or even a lifetime of misery can be avoided.

Same for the adrenals.

Get yourself checked, discuss the results with your doctor, implement any measures to correct any imbalances, and…

get back to being the youthful you and living your life to its full potential.

Stay safe, and may health and happiness be with you wherever you may go.

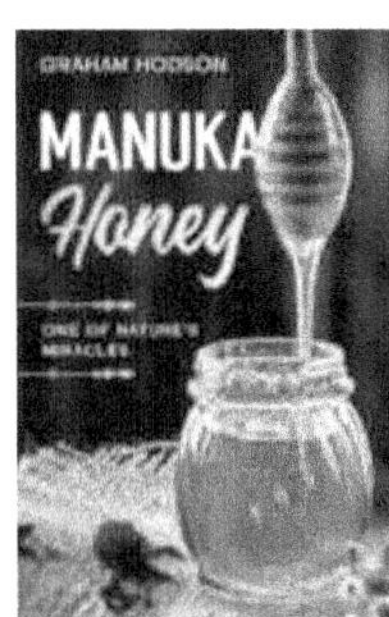
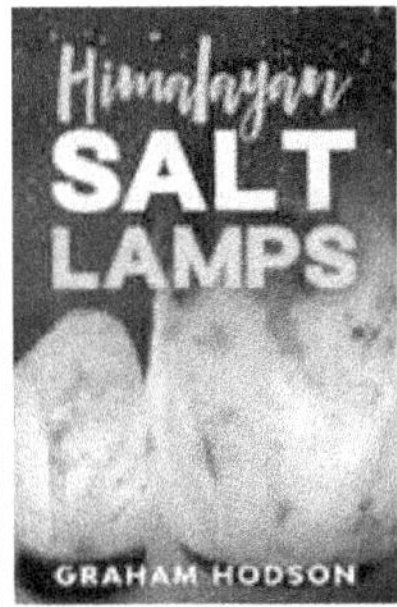
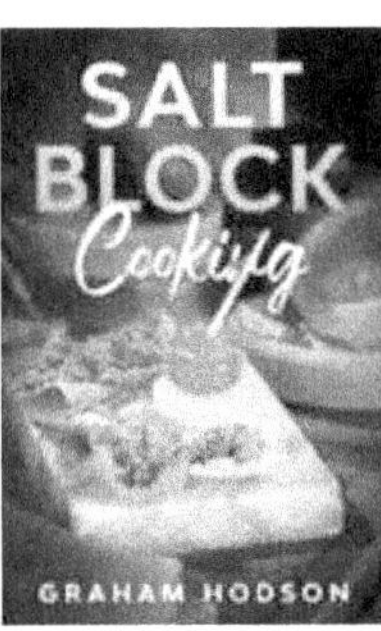
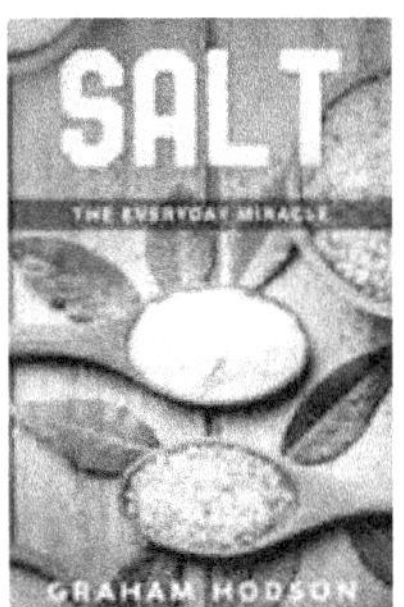
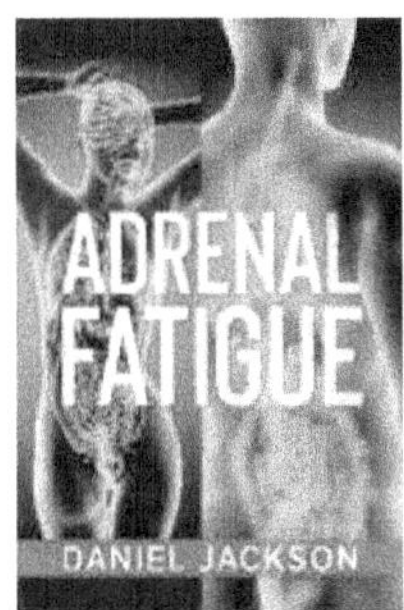
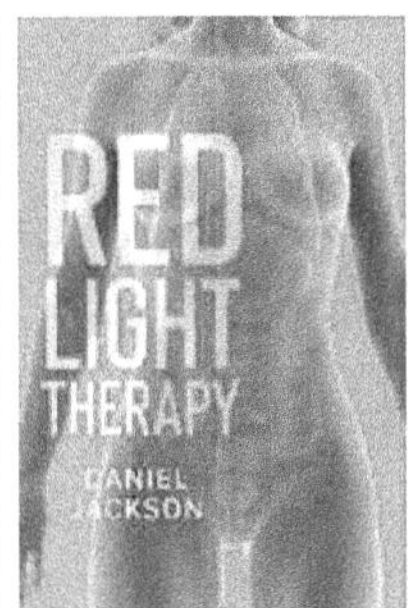
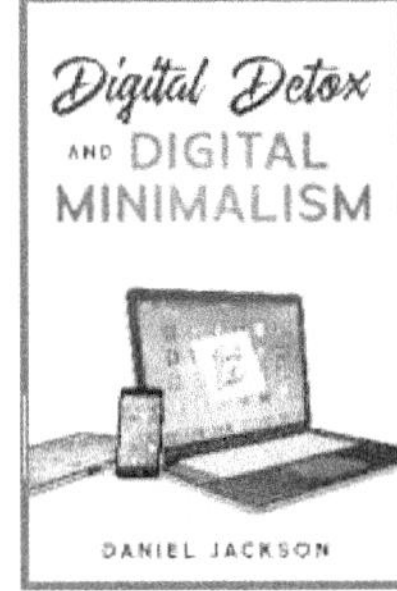
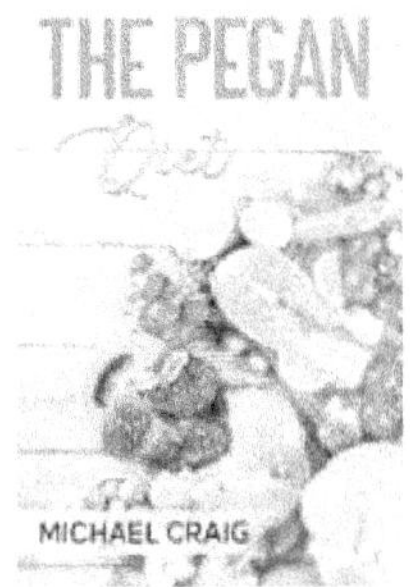

Take a look at more great books available from Rockwood Publishing

… some for FREE!

Just visit the link below:

rockwoodpublishing.co.uk

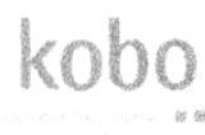
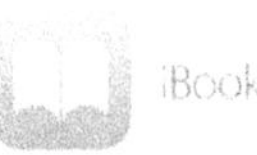
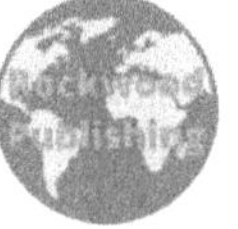
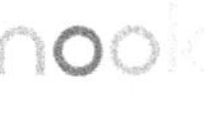
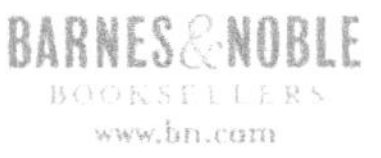

Index

Published by Rockwood Publishing 2021

Copyright and Trademarks. This publication is Copyright 2021 by Rockwood Publishing. All products, publications, software and services mentioned and recommended in this publication are protected by trademarks. In such instances, all trademarks & copyright belong to the respective owners. All rights reserved. No part of this book may be reproduced or transferred in any form or by any means, graphic, electronic, or mechanical, including photocopying, recording, taping, or by any information storage retrieval system, without the written permission of the author. Pictures used in this book are either royalty-free pictures bought from stock-photo websites or have the source mentioned underneath the picture.

Disclaimer and Legal Notice. This product is not legal or medical advice and should not be interpreted in that manner. You need to do your own due diligence to determine if the content of this product is right for you. The author and the affiliates of this product are not liable for any damages or losses associated with the content in this product. While every attempt has been made to verify the information shared in this publication, neither the author nor the affiliates assume any responsibility for errors, omissions or contrary interpretation of the subject matter herein. Any perceived slights to any specific person(s) or organisation(s) are purely unintentional. We have no control over the nature, content and availability of the websites listed in this book. The inclusion of any website links does not necessarily imply a recommendation or endorse the views expressed within them. Rockwood Publishing takes no responsibility for, and will not be liable for, the websites being temporarily unavailable or being removed from the Internet. The accuracy and completeness of the information provided herein and opinions stated herein are not guaranteed or warranted to produce any particular results, and the advice and strategies contained herein may not be suitable for every individual. The author shall not be liable for any loss incurred as a consequence of the use and application, directly or indirectly, of any information presented in this work. This publication is designed to provide information in regards to the subject matter covered. The information included in this book has been compiled to give an overview of the subject(s) and detail some of the symptoms, treatments etc. that are available to people with this condition. It is not intended to give medical advice. For a firm diagnosis of your condition, and for a treatment plan suitable for you, you should consult your doctor or consultant. The writer of this book and the publisher are not responsible for any damages or negative consequences following any of the treatments or methods highlighted in this book. Website links are for informational purposes and should not be seen as a personal endorsement; the same applies to the products detailed in this book. The reader should also be aware that although the web links included were correct at the time of writing, they may become out of date in the future.

Disclaimers

The content contained within this book is for information and entertainment purposes only, and in no way purports to represent professional medical opinion. It should NOT be used as a substitute for expert advice, and you must consult with your designated health professional before acting upon any information contained herein or before undertaking any practice whose methodology is referred to in this book. The author is NOT a registered health professional and the text merely represents personal opinion, not medical fact. The author cannot be held responsible for the consequences of any action derived from the reading of this book, as the content is not based on diagnosis and subsequent regimen. It is the reader's responsibility to seek proper, professional medical advice from a registered health practitioner in connection with any material contained within this book.

Legal Disclaimer (part 1)

Nothing in this book should be construed as an attempt to diagnose, treat or cure. The information in this book is intended to be a community resource. The author takes no responsibility for any informational material or brochures produced using information taken from this book. The author has endeavoured to ensure that all information is correct at the time of publication. This information, however, is subject to change without notice. The author makes no warranty with regard to the accuracy of any information and will not be liable for any errors or omissions. Any liability that arises as a result of this information is hereby excluded to the fullest extent allowed by law.

This information should not be used as a substitute for seeking independent professional advice.

Legal Disclaimer (part 2)

Disclaimer and Terms of Use:

a) i. In publishing this information, the author makes no representations concerning the efficacy, appropriateness or suitability of any products or treatments. Use this information at your own risk. The compiler is not a doctor and has no medical background or training.

ii. Statements and information regarding dietary supplements, books and any products mentioned have not been evaluated by any health authority and are not intended to diagnose, treat, cure or prevent any disease or health condition.

b) In view of the possibility of human error, neither the author nor any other party involved in providing this information, warrant that the information contained therein is in every respect accurate or complete and they are not responsible nor liable for any errors or omissions that may be found or for the results obtained from the use of such information. The entire risk as to the use of this information is assumed by the user.

c) You are encouraged to consult other sources and confirm the information.

d) The information you access is provided "as is". No warranty, expressed or implied, is given as to the accuracy, completeness or timeliness of any information herein, or for obtaining legal advice. To the fullest extent permissible according to applicable law, neither the author nor any other parties who have been involved in the creation, preparation, printing, or delivering of this information assume responsibility for the completeness, accuracy, timeliness, errors or omissions of said information and assume no liability for any direct, incidental, consequential, indirect, or punitive damages as well as any circumstance for any complication, injuries, side effects or other medical accidents to person or property arising from or in connection with the use or reliance upon any information contained herein.

e) The author is not responsible for the contents of any linked site or any link contained in a linked site, or any changes or update to such sites. The inclusion of any link does not imply endorsement by the author. The author makes no representations or claims as to the quality, content and accuracy of the information, services, products, messages which may be provided by such resources, and specifically disclaims any warranties, including but not limited to implied or express warranties of merchantability or fitness for any particular usage, application or purpose.

f) The information provided is general in nature and is intended for educational and informational purposes only. It is not intended to replace or substitute the evaluation, judgment, diagnosis, and medical or preventative care of a physician, paediatrician, therapist and/or health care provider.

g) Any medical, nutritional, dietetic, therapeutic or other decisions, dosages, treatments or drug regimes should be made in consultation with a health care practitioner. Do not discontinue treatment or medication without first consulting your physician, clinician or therapist.

h) By reading this information, you signify your assent to these terms and conditions of use. If you do not agree to these terms and conditions of use, do not read/use this information. If any provision of these terms and conditions of use shall be determined to be unlawful, void or for any reason unenforceable, then that provision shall be deemed severable from this agreement and shall not affect the validity and enforceability of any remaining provisions.

i) The information, services, products, messages and other materials, individually and collectively, are provided with the understanding that the author is not engaged in rendering medical advice or recommendations.

j) The information and the terms of use are subject to change without notice. The material provided as is without warranty of any kind and may include inaccuracies and/or typographical errors. The author makes no representations about the suitability of this information for any purpose. The author disclaims all warranties concerning this information, including all implied warranties, and in no event shall the author be held liable, resulting from, or in any way related to, the use of this information.

k) The unauthorized alteration of the content of this information is expressly prohibited. The author, its agents and representatives shall not be responsible for any claims, actions or damages which may arise on account of the unauthorized alteration of this information.